Table of Contents

Common Indoor Allergies: Triggers, Treatments, and More

1. Introduction to Indoor Allergies

Common indoor allergens include animal dander, dust mite droppings, and cockroach feces, so each space's inhabitants should prioritize those households to prevent indoor allergies. Although children and grandchildren of allergy sufferers are generally more likely to get some type of allergy, the main drivers of allergic diseases are external. In general, home environments with more diverse allergen types are also those with more mixing. Allergens have differing molecular weights and levels of insolubility, and so not all of them travel equally. The allergens that do not penetrate the mucosa will activate our immune system (triggering DNA transcription and the release of T-helper cells, as well as allergy-related cytokines). For all those with sensitization, the symptoms correlate significantly (and most often) with the levels of allergens. Allergic symptoms are very severe where the levels of allergens are highest.

Indoor allergies often contribute to poor health, including lung and skin conditions like eczema, bronchitis, and asthma. In this essay, I cover topics relevant to the causes and effects of common indoor allergens, including trigger sources, allergy genetics, the risk of sensitization across different allergens, allergic responses to certain allergens, prevention and treatment techniques, reasons that allergies develop in the first place, and general trends across studies since the 1900s.

2. Understanding Allergies

At its core, an allergy is the human immune system's response to a substance regarded as likely to cause damage. An allergen is a substance that induces an allergic reaction and can be splintered into multiple categories. Environmental allergens are things such as pollen, outdoor molds, and pet dander. While they may not originate strictly in an indoor environment, people often encounter them inside. Other types of allergens are inherent to indoor living quarters and include everything from dust mites and cockroaches to furry and scaly pets. Food allergies aren't a topic of discussion for this article, for instance, but they're one of the many diverse forms of allergies out there.

Allergies. Hearing the word may make you think of springtime when pollen allergies are in full force. Maybe pet allergies come to mind and you wonder how your friends with pets were able to get the adorable puppy you're so allergic to. The notion of allergies triggering adverse reactions doesn't just apply to outdoor allergens and pets. Indoor environments may contain a multitude of allergens capable of causing allergies, even to those not prone to typical seasonal allergies.

2.1. What Are Allergies?

Basically, allergies are not to be messed with, and there are multiple types of allergies an individual can have. There are many categories that this imaginative response falls under. While allergic reactions, in general, are usually mild or moderate, they can also range from inconveniencing to fatal. Some allergic responses, for example, can be severe enough to cause discoloring of the skin, bad digestive issues, inflamed airways, skin rashes, perturbing odors, and other severe reactions; some frightening enough to get a hefty concern. Many irritating health effects including coughing, dizziness, fatigue, sniffling, sneezing, carpal tunnel, arthritis, multiple sclerosis, fibromyalgia, lupus, vomiting, diarrhea, and itching are some effects that various allergies can have. If a person does not receive necessary medical help in a timely manner, it is indeed possible that individuals may succumb to allergen amounts piling too high on the body.

You may hear people refer to allergies in conversation often, but what are allergies, exactly? Allergies, or allergic diseases, are considered to be a hypersensitivity disorder of the immune system, which is not a disease but just the functioning of the body. Allergic reactions or responses occur when the body's immune system senses and attacks a harmful invader. Many substances make the body produce allergic reactions. The key, however, is whether or not the substance actually triggers a response in the body. Alcoholic beverages, food, food additives, insect venom, latex rubber, medications, metals, and pollens are some common triggers or allergens. It's possible for people of all ages and genders to be affected, and again, these particles are found, can cause, or do cause a reaction on an international or mini level.

2.2. Types of Allergens

The seven types of allergens are: 1. Inhaled - house dust, pollen, mold, dust mites 2. Foods - proteins in cow's milk, wheat, eggs, peanuts, seafood, soy, tree nuts 3. Insect - bee sting venom, insect bites, cockroaches, flies 4. Drug - penicillin, aspirin, ibuprofen, ACE inhibitors, etc. 5. Contact - nickel, latex, poison oak, plants 6. Eye - conjunctivitis 7. Anaphylaxis - severe allergic reaction with symptoms in different body systems

While all allergens can trigger a range of allergic reactions in some individuals, they are classified into a few distinct categories. The presence of these categories can exacerbate someone's allergic tendencies, but each type has different physical manifestations. In the discussion below, we will take a deeper dive into the most common allergens that produce symptoms inside our homes. Allergens are environmental elements that cause an allergic reaction. When inhaled, ingested, or contacted by sensitive individuals, these irritants may cause histamine release and other problems such as coughing, sneezing, or a rash. Component categories include foods, chemical and environmental substances, and pharmaceutical drugs.

3. Common Indoor Allergens

Likewise, those having positive allergy skin tests for a specific allergen are not guaranteed to react to that allergen in real life. A positive skin test for dust mites could only mean that those mites are potential allergenic triggers for that individual. The person needs to be exposed to the specific allergen in the environment and at that time before actual reactions might occur.

Commonality. In the 2003-2006 American National Health and Nutrition Examination Survey, three out of four homes had evidence of cockroach allergens. However, it's uncertain how many produced asthma attacks in affected individuals. In a detail released early access for publication in June 2010, researchers found cockroach allergens in up to 82 percent of urban homes have been associated with increased risk for asthma. However, it's also been impossible to predict individual cockroach exposure, in part due to variability in patients' housing and other factors.

Specificity. In some situations, people react to only one allergy-triggering parameter, but others have multiple problems that often overlap. Also, sometimes allergies trigger other allergies, such as eczema.

There are plenty of substances that stir up trouble in people prone to allergies, and many of the allergens are found inside. In this essay, you will learn more about the most common ones and the potential impact they have on your health. First, however, it's important to understand the basic characteristics of the allergens to which you might be reacting.

3.1. Dust Mites

The feces and dead skin patches from these mites trigger an allergic reaction in some people. Keys to managing dust mite allergies include removing their sources and avoiding getting rid of their waste. More serious cases may require medications or additional treatments that help avoid allergic symptoms from forming.

Dust mites are tiny insects that cover our bodies and can be found in the tiniest nooks and crannies of the home. Although they are a common problem in homes, they are not as common in plants, unlike many other insects that are considered pests. Dust mites consume flakes of human skin, which fall off and can be found in the hair or even in your pillow. Exasperating for those with dust mite allergies, these bugs are found in every location of the home: the dust created by air conditioning units is just as probable of a home for these mites as under the couch.

Indoor allergens are substances that cause allergic reactions (like sneezing or watery eyes). There are a few common indoor allergens that cause allergies and asthma to flare. A typical household pet might not seem all that threatening at first. However, for those with household allergies, exposure to pet dander (among other things) can be quite uncomfortable. This article delves into three of the most common indoor allergens—including pet dander.

3.2. Pet Dander

Many people believe that pet fur is an allergen, but it is not. The dander and the proteins that stick to the fur are the real triggers for most people who are allergic to cats or dogs. As a result, while it's important to keep our pets clean and brushed to keep the dander from sticking to them, removing the source of the dander—your pet—is virtually the only form of allergy treatment that won't just mask the symptoms. If you're allergic to a pet, you know how undesirable the reaction can be. Symptoms include itchy, watering eyes, runny nose, coughing, wheezing, and sneezing. If you're determined to remain a pet owner, you'll wish to seek out the assistance of an specialist who can suggest appropriate treatments.

Pet Dander Strictly speaking, pet dander isn't only the small, round epithelial cells we (or more accurately, they) shed as part of our hair and skin renewal. It is also made up of saliva and urine proteins, which can stick to the hair and feathers as the animals groom themselves. These proteins mix with whatever allergens the pet has to pick up from the world around them, such as dust mites or pollen. The dander and airborne urine are then inhaled by those who live in close contact with the pet.

Now, we'll take a closer look at what pet dander is and how it can trigger indoor allergies.

3.3. Mold

Symptoms of allergic rhinitis caused by mold particles include a stuffy or runny nose, sneezing, itchy eyes, and asthma symptoms. The symptoms of mold allergies can overlap with symptoms caused by pet dander, dust mites, and ragweed. The American College of Allergy, Asthma and Immunology lists some symptoms that could differentiate mold allergies from other similar respiratory conditions. People with a mold allergy may experience prolonged asthma symptoms, especially whenever the weather is damp, mold exposure is high, or when they are in a damp or moldy place. Unlike the symptoms that usually occur with hay fever (allergic rhinitis) every fall, people with mold allergies may experience symptoms at any time. For people who are sensitive and allergic to mold, avoid living in damp, dark, poorly ventilated, and moldy places. This could include old or poorly constructed homes, closets, or garages. Furthermore, since allergy shots can be helpful in reducing symptoms in certain people, for severe mold allergy symptoms, seek support from an allergist.

Mold is another common indoor allergen. It's a type of fungus that grows in damp, dim conditions with poor air circulation. Despite the name, mold isn't only associated with food spoilage; it can also be found indoors on fabric, paper, wood, and other materials. The musty smell often associated with "moldy" environments is due to the volatile organic compounds released by some species of molds. Molds spread by producing large numbers of small, lightweight spores that can travel through the air. Some molds produce hazardous mycotoxins. A 2004 review published in the journal Toxicology and Industrial Health reported that indoor air concentrations of a variety of molds were directly correlated with both the crustal incidence of respiratory symptoms and poor lung function. Inflammatory reactions to a high mold spore load or mold toxins can cause lung damage.

3.4. Cockroaches

The scary news is that living with cockroach allergens –
especially in the newborn to 2-year-old set – is actually
risky. Desensitizing the kids doesn't seem to work as well,
nor does desensitizing their caregivers. More importantly,
the extent of airborne cockroach allergen inside homes is
thought to show how bad the life of the cockroaches living
in the home actually is. Therefore, a positive test to an
indoor-specific cockroach allergen is a likely sign that there
are still a lot of cockroaches in the house you're living in,
and therefore an increased risk can be substantial. After all,
if there are any indoor cockroaches, there is probably some
good-sized water source around too.

Every time you talk about indoor allergens, you are sure to
be hearing about dust mites. News flash: roaches are a way
bigger deal when it comes to causing allergies. Although
the majority of common American roaches do not live
indoors, there are some that exclusively live indoors
(therefore, very urban). If you have cockroaches, you need
to exterminate them! Ideally, you should call an
exterminator who knows how to get rid of cockroaches in a
way that doesn't spread pesticides around your living
space. Often, if you live in any type of rental property, the
penalty for spreading cockroaches around the building far
exceeds the benefit of getting rid of the bugs. Yelling at the
kids doesn't help either, you need an expert. Rules to live
by – wipe up food crumbs, do not leave pet food sitting
around, do not leave dishes in the sink. If you seriously
have cockroaches, no excuses for leaving dishes out.

4. Symptoms of Indoor Allergies

It is important to be able to recognize the symptoms of common indoor allergies and realize possible causes when an individual is suffering from them. When in doubt, consult with your healthcare professional. One of the most common signs of indoor allergies is a stuffy nose. Rhinitis, the inflammation of the lining of the nasal passages, is mainly characterized by excessive mucus production, causing a stuffy nose. The excessive mucus production is courtesy of the nasal passages attempting to wash away and eliminate dust and other allergy triggers, such as pet hair and dander, that the individual has inhaled. As the nasal passages become swollen from an allergic reaction, it can hamper the person's sense of smell. An individual with chronic rhinitis may also develop chronic sinusitis. As the nasal passages become swollen and obstructed due to the chronic rhinitis, the sinuses can no longer drain properly. The trapped mucus is a perfect breeding ground for bacteria. Symptoms of chronic sinusitis include excessively thick mucus, nasal blockage, headaches, and facial pain or tenderness. Other common indoor allergies include most common respiratory and skin symptoms.

Some common respiratory symptoms of indoor allergies include coughing, sneezing, and a nasal drip. Some individuals may also experience a decrease in their ability to smell. Those with asthma may also have an asthma attack after breathing in the trigger or triggers. Other respiratory-related signs and symptoms of indoor allergies include wheezing or a tight feeling in the chest. Some people may also experience generalized fatigue or irritability. In addition to respiratory symptoms, indoor allergens can also cause people to develop skin symptoms, such as itching and/or hives and eczema.

In other words, respiratory symptoms are most of what affects the way we breathe. There are a number of specific disorders that make up the element of breathing called respiratory symptoms. The ones associated with indoor allergens include allergic rhinitis and its subtypes and "allergic" forms of sinusitis, cough, bronchitis, and bronchial asthma. Nasal allergy is also called allergic rhinitis, and it includes specific forms with and without nasal polyps. The nasal passages are often referred to as your "nose," and the sinus cavities are often called the "paranasal sinuses" or "sinuses." The lower airway is a loose, much-branched, air-filled tube that connects your windpipe to your deeper lungs, and it is the source of feedback to our sensory nervous system that regulates the amount of air we breathe in and out each minute.

Life is incredibly different when you have to deal with respiratory symptoms every day. The most common respiratory complaint is a stuffy nose. Other respiratory symptoms include frequent episodes of: - Sneezing. - Itchy nose, throat, or roof of mouth. - Symptoms of sinus infection, such as facial pressure or headache, stuffy/congested nose, or decreased sense of smell. - Multiple episodes of coughing or a lasting cough. - Shortness of breath, chest tightness, or wheezing.

4.1. Respiratory Symptoms

Common indoor allergies

4.2. Skin Symptoms

Skin symptoms If left untreated, indoor allergens can cause a variety of skin symptoms. Itchy skin, which is also known as pruritus, can occur anywhere on the body. The itching can be more severe in locations where a person was bitten by a biting insect. It may be difficult to think about skin without thinking about our hair. However, facial itching can also occur. Itching can be especially uncomfortable around the eyes. Swelling can develop where there is itching due to indoor allergies. Hives, also called welts, can be seen as raised, red, itchy, and irregularly shaped bumps in the areas of the skin that have been exposed to an indoor allergen. Hives can appear and disappear quickly and can move around. Skin may be excessively dry with indoor allergens. A classic example is when the skin is dry due to contact with a wool sweater. People with indoor allergies may notice that their skin is drier than normal during an allergic reaction.

Where do indoor allergies come from? Millions of people suffer from indoor allergies. The severity of allergic symptoms can range from mild to severe. Some of the most common allergens that cause reactions are usually found indoors. There are many things that can cause indoor allergies, and most of them are a small insect called a dust mite. Dust mites live indoors and mainly eat skin cells. Household pets and mold are the other common causes of indoor allergies. These are only a few examples of the many possible sources of indoor allergies.

5. Diagnosis of Indoor Allergies

The only way you can find out what allergens will affect you indoors or out is to go to an allergist and get Clinical provocation Testing. An allergist is a physician specially trained to manage and treat allergies, asthma and the other allergic diseases. Call your local allergy association for a list of allergists close to you. The two-part testing includes a skin test and an RAST Test. The skin test or prick test is highly accurate, relatively painless and instant. The intradermal skin test penetrates the skin and is ideal for identifying allergies like insect bites, mold, pet dander and dust mites. Identifying where the allergic reactions occur on the skin signals the doctor as to what category the allergy falls into (four categories of allergies including; Inhalant, Foods and Additives, Perfumed Additives and Chemicals, and Environmental). Each of these four categories has its own specific treatment. An elevated total serum IgE levels (RAST Test) may be observed particularly for those allergic to house dust mites or molds. The RAST Test is a simple blood test that can be performed even if the patient is experiencing an acute allergic skin rash and may even be off medication.

AD - rods and a test strip. You now have to be tested for at least twelve different medications over a several day period until you can learn what you are allergic to and what medications you can take. Dermatology testing has improved, and so has food allergy testing. But the rest of the allergies are essentially the same as they were 30 years ago. An ever-growing population of hay fever sufferers seems to grow every year, and the fact that you can only be tested for what they can accurately diagnose. There are other diagnostic allergy tests but they are very time-consuming and not all need to be done. Serums can be customized if you have been tested with another company, but the person who treats the allergies should always try the company they are most familiar with and have the most confidence using.

5.1. Medical History and Physical Examination

Physical Signs in the Nose - The physical examination is focused on the nose to look for pale mucosa (bluish gray mucosa), thin and watery rhinorrhea, cobblestone mucosa as well as frequent sneezing or nasal "salute". The cue-looking patient may exhibit Shiner's, a blackish discoloration under the eyes, or a glazed appearance to the eyes with Dennie-Morgan lines at the lower lid margin. Examine the lips for eczema, referred to as "lick and rub" or "allergic salute". Itching of the Ears - The patient may complain of itching of the inner ear, chronic ear infections, or a "clogged" inner ear. People who chronically finger or rub their ears are considered by some to be at higher risk for the development of chronic sinusitis (inner ear inflammation). Paleness and/or blue/grayish or swollen lower eyelid with Dennie-Morgan infraorbital fold may be noted bilaterally in the "allergic shiner". Regular upward rubbing against the nose often will produce an allergic crease across the nostrils of the patient.

Initial diagnosis of IA is made by collecting a thorough medical history and conducting a complete physical examination. Health care providers must have a general understanding of the patient's lifestyle and living conditions, as well as their reaction to common allergens present in the homes of the general population, in order to correctly initiate the IA diagnostic process. It is helpful to discuss the specific allergens such as pet dander, various molds, dust mites, and roaches, to which individual patients might be allergic. How to avoid the infrequent allergens found in work or educational settings will depend on the patient's occupation and place of employment. It is necessary to identify causative allergens in the symptomatic patient in order to accomplish thorough avoidance. Additional diagnostic testing is warranted to confirm the diagnosis of IA and identify the relevant allergen(s). Indications for testing include individual patient's resources, degree of daily function that is compromised by symptoms, impact on quality of life, and need to document the diagnosis of IA for possible benefit in the legal arena. It should be pointed out to patients that tests for IA are often negative if they have used full doses of antihistamines right up to the allergy test.

Section 5.1: Medical History and Physical Examination

5.2. Allergy Testing

Skin Prick Test A skin prick test involves placing liquid extracts of the allergens on the skin and pricking the skin to see if the body has an immediate or delayed reaction. A control test is also performed, as each person may react in different ways. The control is often performed with histamine (the body's own chemical that produces allergy symptoms), and the other test uses sterile saline solution as a negative control. Measurement of the reaction is then performed at 15 minutes for an immediate reaction and then again from 48 hours to as long as a week to see if a 'delayed' reaction will occur. More recently, there are newly developed antihistamine and steroid creams that the allergist can use to block the allergic effects of histamine and to decrease the swelling (inflammation) that occurs with the delayed 'prick' test.

An allergy test is an important part of diagnosing indoor allergies. There are multiple ways this test can be performed. The skin prick test is the most common form of allergy testing. It typically takes place on the forearm but can also be performed on the upper back. This testing does involve needles, but they do not go in extremely deep. Common results can be produced in as little as 15 to 20 minutes. They are typically diagnosed by an allergic disease specialist. Other methods of allergy testing include blood tests and patch tests which do not require needles.

6. Managing Indoor Allergies

Reducing allergens at home proved to be beneficial for asthmatic patients sensitized to mites. In general, it could not be shown that a pets-are-forbidden rule changes the frequency of sensitization at an early age. All subjects should be adequately informed about the allergen avoiding methods that are recommended because they are efficient. Data show that it is possible to prevent development of sensitization to perennial allergens as well as asthma by reducing the level of mite allergens. Prevention cannot be supposed to be active if the subject was sensitized to the allergens. Mitigation of exposure became a coadjuvant therapy to reduce the intensity and sensitivity of the allergic inflammation in sensitized patients, and probably to prevent the development of other allergies.

Treatment of indoor allergies aims to limit exposure to indoor allergens in combination with alleviating allergic symptoms when they do peak. It is rather challenging to reduce animal dander in homes that have pets. Lacking complete allergen eradication, additional strategies become necessary. These strategies can be divided into allergen avoidance and symptomatic relief. For mites, it is recommended to truly avoid contact with the mite by using special mattress and pillow coverings. Mite allergens in mattresses and higher concentrations of pet dander lead to allergic symptoms. Condensation and growth of mites is limited if encasings are pure. The patient must be well informed that encasings need to be used for a long term, since allergen levels decrease slowly.

Dust mites: Mattress cases and pillow encasings can be purchased at discount department stores and bedding stores. There are several manufacturers that sell dust mite-impermeable covers for mattresses, pillows, and box springs. Newer covers are made of smooth, slippery fabrics that are more comfortable and less likely to hold moisture under the host's body weight. You must use mite-impermeable pup-proof covers which zip snugly around the mattress and completely encase the pillow, box spring, and comforter. High-efficiency air filters, although relatively pricey, are available for heating and cooling systems temporarily. HEPA filters do not require replacement, allowing for limitless use. The addition of a pleated high-efficiency air filter can complement an electronic air cleaner for those suffering from sinusitis, allergies, or asthma. Use moist cloths with water or your choice of polish to dust wood furniture, baseboards, beams, wainscotting, etc. To dust frames and low shelves, use a slightly damp cloth. Dust exterior window sills, ledges, storm windows, and window frames. Regularly polish wood to discourage dust accumulation. Dust toys while they are clean with soapy water. If practical, use a high-efficiency vacuum cleaner that uses HEPA filtration. Restrict the activity of the vacuum. Consider using a consultant or company that specializes in allergy-proofing your house. If a good candidate for therapy, avoiding listed pets in the home can be considered. If you vacuum the home, consider removing allergen-containing rugs; if you are covering an existing carpet. The person allergic to pets should stay away from pets, pet dander, and pet skin scales.

If you are allergic to an indoor allergen, the most important step in your environmental control program is to eliminate or minimize your contact with that allergen as much as possible. Your physician and/or allergist can help you identify strategies that are most appropriate for your individual situation.

6.2. Medications

Antihistamines block histamine's movement to histaminic receptors, preventing certain people from experiencing a histamine response. In the United States, antihistamine medications are now available OTC. Second-generation antihistamines are preferred to first-generation antihistamines. Although some users may feel drowsy, most second-gen antihistamines appear to be reasonably effective. Histamine-induced swelling, itchiness, and mucus manufacture are all diminished by leukotriene inhibitors.

Leukotriene receptor antagonists (LTRAs) are taken in medication form and are used to reduce swelling and relax the airways. Also referred to as leukotriene modifiers, montelukast (Singulair) is the most popular of the LTRAs.

In contrast to the short-acting beta-agonists typically used to alleviate acute asthma symptoms, ICS help reduce and manage allergic inflammation of the lungs. INCS, like their nasal version, have anti-inflammatory properties and can help alleviate diseases associated with indoor allergies.

INCS medications are available as a generic and over the counter (OTC). Fluticasone propionate (Flonase) is the most common INCS drug available OTC. Those who experience wheezing in conjunction with their allergies might profit from inhaled corticosteroids.

Numerous medications can be taken alone or combined to alleviate symptoms resulting from indoor allergies. Intranasal corticosteroids (INCS) are commonly used to treat respiratory allergies. These anti-inflammatory medications reduce congestion, nasal itchiness, sneezing, and other symptoms. Unlike oral medications, INCS have a delayed onset of action of 12 to 24 hours. Full use is recommended for better results. Seasonal rhinitis sufferers willing to tolerate nasal sprays should begin using their medication several days before symptoms arise.

6.3. Immunotherapy

It is a form of treatment against the causative agents of allergic diseases, rather than treating allergy symptoms with daily medications and should be considered in individuals with a reliable clinical diagnosis, whose symptoms do not respond well to regular treatment and who have been shown to be allergic to one or more indoor allergens and have tested with skin-prick tests or in vitro tests to be specific to that trigger. They are also contraindicated in poor or noncompliant individuals. Immunotherapy generally is a long-term treatment, with the build-up phase taking about three to six months, followed by a maintenance phase that typically lasts between three and five years. Successful completion of this treatment can result in lasting relief from allergy symptoms, sometimes even after treatment stops.

Patients with allergic rhinitis and/or asthma by aeroallergens from house dust mites or probably indoor pets can benefit from immunotherapy which specifically targets the underlying cause, and allergist/immunologists have enormous experience using this therapy.

Immunotherapy, or allergy shots, is one of the outstanding features of modern allergy care and management. Modern immunotherapy was first introduced in the early twentieth century but has mostly gained traction in the more recent period. Broadly speaking, there are two types of immunotherapy: subcutaneous and sublingual. In subcutaneous immunotherapy, allergens are injected under the skin with a specific schedule to initiate and maintain the "immunologic tolerance." On the other hand, in sublingual immunotherapy, which is relatively more convenient, the patient treats himself or herself with drops that are taken in daily dosing directly under their tongues for the same purpose as subcutaneous injection to avoid the way of the tolerance.

7. Creating an Allergy-Friendly Home

9. Keep pests out. Store food in airtight containers, seal cracks and holes, and put trash in a bin with a lid.

8. Use machines with air filters. An air purifier with a high-efficiency particulate air (HEPA) filter can help capture particles that trigger allergy symptoms. HEPA-covered cooling and heating systems help keep outdoor allergens from circulating inside.

7. Use a vacuum cleaner with a high-efficiency particulate air (HEPA) filter. The vacuum cleaner's powerful suction and efficient filter will work in tandem to lift hidden dirt, pet dander, and other potential respiratory irritants from deep within the carpet and capture those particles in its filter rather than allowing them to be redistributed back into the indoor air.

6. Dust cloth storage. Many homeowners already have a few microfiber dust cloths in their cleaning arsenal. However, these materials can actually draw in dust mites, distribute them around the house when dusting, and allow residual mites to thrive in the fibers.

5. Use allergy-friendly products. From cleaning products and laundry detergent to scent diffusers and cleaning sponges, many of our shopping purchases can hold surprise allergens that could be impacting our respiratory health. When shopping for cleaning products, look for gentle yet effective options.

4. Get rid of clutter. This includes items like knickknacks that gather dust and can be difficult to clean. Opt for simple, washable decor.

3. Try hardwood or laminate flooring. Avoid wall-to-wall carpeting.

2. Regularly clean pet habitats. Clean cages and litter boxes often, and make sure your pets spend time in rooms where you're not sleeping.

1. Close windows and doors. Keep doors and windows closed to prevent pollen and outdoor mold from coming inside.

The aim of an allergy-friendly home is to create a living space that minimizes exposure to indoor allergens like pet dander, dust mites, mold, and insects. If you have allergies or asthma, the home environment can play a large role in your overall health. Use these strategies to manage your or your family's indoor allergies:

Allergy-Friendly Homes

7.1. Cleaning Tips

For most people, cleaning may be the last thing that you
would spin your heels over. Dusters, mops, brooms, and
vacuums have taken on new importance since the last time
we took a good, hard look at our homes. To help alleviate
allergies, asthma, or hay fever for the home, consider the
following particular cleaning strategies. Dust mites love to
appear on surfaces in every room of your home which
come into contact with the human body. These might
include mattresses, pillows, under beds or sofas, and
carpets. Dust mites are also attracted to soft textures, so
they may also be in objects like soft toys, upholstered
furniture, curtains, and other linens. Consider these
specific tips for how to get rid of these contaminants.

For the most allergy-friendly homes, it's all about
cleanliness. Begin by making the bed, properly covering
sleep encasements and re-washing and drying the top
bedding. Make sure comforters are machine washable, and
sheets are machine washable and allergist. Wash laundry
at least once weekly using a high-efficiency (HE) machine
and detect detergent marked "fragrance-free." Using cold
water and hot drying cycles can help kill dust mites and
their eggs locking into fabric fibers. An allergist exhausts
fan out of the house or cover with a non-allergen grill to
keep moist air from circulating indoors, and ensure that
the vent is working properly when steam is lingering in the
bathroom.

7.2. Ventilation and Air Filtration

Air naturals are small particles that are derived from proteins of a variety of mammalian species. These proteins are found in the skin, urine, saliva, and feces of most orders of animals. Once imposed inside a home, we can breathe in this protein and trigger an allergic reaction. The most common culprits are dogs, cats, gerbils, and rabbits. Animal dander can also stick to dust mites and pollen in your house. That's why pet allergens can still be found in households after the pet has long left. Common indoor allergens are small particles that consist of the shed skin cells of humans and animals. These flakes are so tiny that they can be inhaled straight into the lungs when carpets are walked or furniture is shaken. Each of us emits about 100 grams of skin flakes a week. These skin flakes are contaminated by a protein found in most people which triggers allergies. Pets also have specific proteins that in some individuals can trigger allergies.

Ventilation is the intentional flow of outdoor air indoors. This is mainly accomplished through windows, doors, and vents within the building. This process can help reduce indoor air pollutants by replacing contaminated air indoors with fresh outdoor air. On the other hand, effective air filtration can remove up to 99.7 percent of airborne particles. The use of an air purifier can reduce allergens in the air, such as pet dander, mold spores, dust, and pollen. However, this does not have any effect on allergens that are in haystacks and upholstery. If an air purifier is combined with other prevention strategies, it can be a helpful part of an allergy management plan.

8. Indoor Allergies in Specific Populations

In the medical and scientific literature, much of which covers both children and adults, limited data regarding the prevalence and influence of allergies in the elderly exist. Because of differences in pediatric and adult factors, however, the issue of allergies and incidence in the elderly may not transfer to the pediatric population. Reduced immune sensitivities, age-related inflammation, and pathophysiological processes place older adults at a lesser risk of an allergic reaction than their younger counterparts. Solid clinical vaccine therapy data, meanwhile, suggest that the protection of older persons against vaccine challenges is both poor and not durable. Older individuals with allergies have similar allergic symptoms to the same source of allergens as other age groups. However, general age-related conditions such as existing treatments, medication administration, or concurrent infections can obscure allergy signs and further link allergic symptoms possibly to older individuals' solitary or multiple clinical conditions. In general, the symptoms of allergic upper respiratory illness are mild in older adults, with reduced asthma occurrence and airway hyperresponsiveness compared to older individuals without allergies.

Indoor allergies in the elderly

Their developing respiratory systems account for children's increased susceptibility to indoor allergens and related complications. Given their increased frequency outdoors and increased exposure to indoor allergens such as pet dander and dust mites, more severe allergic reactions in children are not uncommon. Even older individuals can have indoor allergies, whether or not they are first-time parents and have not had any allergies before. Mildew is a fungal spore that grows in damp areas of a child's respiratory system, natural carpeting, and bedding, and can cause sinus infections, colds, and other respiratory problems, in worst cases. Moreover, allergy effects in youngsters coughing and wheezing can trigger puffing assaults before allergy symptoms appear. When children sneeze and cough, they indicate the presence of other microbial respiratory infections. Colds with swollen nasal passages and a gooey nose can develop symptoms of respiratory allergies to meet mild symptoms in adults, and vice versa. Because no one knows how they'll adjust to climate change. Because indoor allergens are year-round nuisances, some persons could continue to have an increasing incidence of allergies.

Indoor allergies for children

8.1. Children

Many of the same tips that help adults manage their indoor allergies can be helpful in managing indoor allergies in children. It is important to help your child avoid their specific allergy triggers. You should identify indoor allergens that may affect your child and take steps to reduce your child's exposure to these triggers. Common pediatric indoor allergy triggers include dust mites, pet dander, mold, and pollen. Environmental controls, including the use of bedding and pillow covers that are designed to limit exposure to dust mites, can help reduce the incidence of childhood allergic diseases. It may also be helpful to invest in an indoor air purifier, as well as carpets that are specifically designed to limit exposure to common household allergens. If possible, remove wall-to-wall carpets from your home altogether. Keep surfaces in your home as clean as possible. Use wet cloths or mops when possible, as dry wipes can release dust back into the air.

Dealing with allergies is already challenging, but addressing the same symptoms in children requires an added level of care. Many of the treatment options that are available today are only recommended for children ages 6 and older. Several over-the-counter and prescription allergy medications are safe for use by children 6 years and older, but many people prefer to explore other options to reduce their children's need for allergy medications.

Children can suffer from many of the same common indoor allergens that affect adults. However, addressing these symptoms in children has its own specific considerations.

8.2. Elderly Individuals

When considering the elderly, like many young children, the common cold is not a limitless energy consumer. While elderly people have congested sinuses, therapeutic options are more challenging. Those who opt for surgery may face increased chances of complication during general anesthesia or risk of complications under general anesthesia, such as myocardial infarction or death. Older people attend hospitals and emergency departments for asthma more than inpatient settings. In the outpatient settings in New York, the hospitalization rate for older adults is 15-30% versus 3-5% for the general population. Only 20% of older adults with asthma suffer from allergic reactiveness using subjective tests of self-reporting. Non-allergic asthma may have an oral or inhaled steroid taper or a pulmonary steroid taper strategy. Systemic steroids used to target the whole body are recommended to limit, reduce, or halt an inflammatory process. Alternate-day oral prednisone for at least 12 weeks, then a reduction over 12-24 months if no adverse reactions to the low dosage (typically 5-10 mg/day) or inhaled corticosteroids over 3-4 weeks to prevent harm to adrenal gland functioning.

The impact of indoor allergies on an aging population is substantial. This segment of the population may be times more in number than children with asthma. Health experts have tended to focus on children because of asthma's interplay with the lungs' natural growth and development time of the airways, among other reasons. Yet, impacts to other older populations, older adults of allergy and its close ties to asthma, may be significant. Experts know that seniors are at higher risk of combining several diseases or "having a great deal of multimorbidity". They may suffer from depression, incontinence, physical inactivity, and social isolation from the loss of a spouse or children moving out of the community.

9. The Link Between Indoor Allergies and Asthma

Regardless, indoor allergen exposure, research suggests, can contribute to triggering allergic reactions and asthma symptoms. These allergens can lead to the development of asthma via a series of responses that compromise the ability to breathe clearly. When a person encounters an allergen to which their immune system is allergic, they experience an overreaction. This overreaction, which is also called sensitization, causes the release of chemicals, such as an antibody known as immunoglobulin E (IgE), and the histamine from immune system cells. The IgE antibodies help our bodies remember this allergen and prompt the next response to the allergen. Immune system cells also release inflammatory substances that can cause swelling in airways (known as inflammation) makes their walls even more irritable or twitchy. This can lead to an asthma episode. Approximately 60% of people have cat allergen in their house (courtesy of cats, other pets, or on the clothing of people who have pets). Even if the individual removes the pets, the allergen can remain up to 8 months. Cats can make even larger amounts of this potent allergen if they are not spayed/neutered.

According to the American Academy of Allergy, Asthma & Immunology (AAAAI), about 75% of individuals in the United States with asthma are allergic to at least one inhalant (indoor) allergen. Core indoor allergens include dust mites, pet dander, mold spores, and/or insect droppings. Although someone with an allergy isn't guaranteed to develop asthma, research suggests they do have a higher risk of doing so than those without allergies. Similarly, asthma risk may be lower in children who didn't develop allergies to common allergens, such as cat dander and dust mites, after they were born.

10. Conclusion and Future Directions

In the next ten years, the main clinical, epidemiological and experimental approaches are expected to provide a better understanding of these issues on the links between the environment and allergic diseases. In a clinical approach, it is essential to continue the study of the in vitro and in vivo tools currently used in the diagnosis and follow-up of allergy to develop, standardize and study new methods for this purpose. Although in vitro methods are preferred to investigate IgE production in humans, these models cannot fully replace the study of human tissues difficult, and the study of IgE production of histamine cells obtained from in vitro umbilical cord blood could provide important evidence in humans. This will facilitate our studies' translation into human diseases, and although several advances about the roles of "B cells", and consequently of IgE, in inflammatory and resident allergic cells have been achieved, this problem requires further investigation. In addition, in other cell types such as "basophils" or mast cells, "calcineurin inhibitors" and "B lymphocyte stimulators" are being studied to reduce synthesis of IgE and "basophil activation patterns" or "histamine release test", respectively. It is also important to identify early allergic markers, such as eosinophilia or neutrophilia following in vitro re-exposures of peripheral blood mononuclear cells to allergen. Detection of atopic diseases is still an important approach in humans. Given the rise in food allergies as well and their close association with rhinoconjunctivitis and asthma, in addition to food intake history, allergic history, prick tests, monitoring and food challenges, the response to humoral IgE often shows a serious impact on the diagnosis and monitoring in the future. In this context, it could follow-up on the effect of anti-IgE on different cells. In future-pragmatic experimental studies, we expect further research on i) the release of metabolites of "eosinophils" in lung allergic diseases and the establishment of "in vitro" methods to investigate the impact of inhaled medications, such as "phytotherapy", "glucocorticosteroids" or "Leukotriene receptor antagonists" on "eosinophils", particularly in humans. These research approaches have already provided new evidence suggesting the potential anti-allergic effects of non-corticosteroids and the possible similarities between allergic lung diseases and asthma in humans to mice.

In conclusion, increased environmental exposure to indoor allergens may be associated with an increased risk of developing allergic diseases, including allergic asthma and rhinoconjunctivitis. Additionally, environmental risk factors for sensitization could be gender or other individual sex markers, maternal age, and geographic location. These observations are possible new research directions for study. Finally, the strategies for the management and reduction of indoor environmental allergens, although not known, are necessary for managing patients with high-risk allergies of this nature, including pregnant women, subscribers to assisted reproductive technologies, children with asthma, children with an allergic background or siblings of ongoing atopic children. To minimize the potential cross-sectional risk of indoor allergies in all patients, avoiding or removing allergen sources should be considered. The long-term result of those strategies to evaluate the development of allergic diseases that have potential damage is feasible when feasible; special attention should be administered to those allergic to early stages to global allergens and pregnant women with a positive maternal history (MPH of allergic diseases).

Effective Strategies for Managing Indoor Allergy Triggers

1. Introduction to Indoor Allergy Triggers

Here, Let's Talk Science is going to present information on indoor allergy triggers to create a better understanding of these common triggers and their prevalence. By understanding the main allergy triggers and how to effectively manage them, we can hope to prevent or reduce exposure and, consequently, mitigate their health impact.

The American College of Allergy, Asthma, and Immunology (AAAAI) reports that allergic asthma is the most common type of asthma. It occurs when the body's immune system responds to a specific allergen in the environment such as pet hair, dust mite, or cockroach droppings. The allergen triggers an inflammatory response in the lungs, which leads to coughing, wheezing, shortness of breath, and chest tightness. Therefore, to reduce the risk of developing allergic diseases, control measures such as improving indoor air quality are often recommended.

Indoor allergens are anything in the environment that provoke an allergic reaction, triggering the release of histamines and other chemicals that lead to sneezing, wheezing, itching, and other uncomfortable symptoms. Common indoor allergens include pet dander and hair, secondhand smoke, cockroaches and other pests, mold spores, and house dust. According to the Centers for Disease Control and Prevention (CDC), more than 50% of people in the US test positive for one or more allergies, which can make managing indoor allergies even more challenging.

1.1. Common Indoor Allergens

Many studies have revealed that indoor allergens can have widely different physical characteristics. The allergens found in dust mite, pet dander, and cockroach are all derived from minuscule sources that are capable of becoming airborne. In addition, the allergens from these sources can travel or be spread via pathways or carry-off mechanisms to other rooms in our homes. When dealing with these allergens, it is important to determine the characteristic of each allergen present, as these properties determine some of the strategies that can help control allergens and improve the indoor environment. The section below addresses the nature of the most common indoor allergens, like from pets and pests, mold spores, and dust mites, and where they can be found.

Our indoor environment can harbor many different kinds of allergens that, when inhaled or touched, can trigger unpleasant symptoms in those who are allergic. Common indoor allergens include dust mites, pet dander (from fur, skin or feathers), cockroach droppings, and mold spores. These allergens are frequently encountered in carpets, upholstery, and bedding, as well as other floor coverings (like wood flooring) and porous wall surfaces in our homes. Compared to the outdoor allergens to which we are exposed, indoor allergens are found in fairly high concentrations due to their indoor environments in our homes and workplaces. As a result, when exposed, those who are allergic to these allergens are likely to experience bothersome symptoms of an allergic reaction every day of the year.

1.2. Symptoms of Indoor Allergies

The skin can also be affected by indoor allergies. Rashes, hives, eczema (atopic dermatitis), and contact dermatitis are examples of skin reactions that may occur. Skin reactions may result from contact with an allergen either by direct physical contact or by exposure to allergens in the air. Repetitive contact or association with an allergen is required to produce skin inflammation. This is why folliculitis or acne is not caused by allergies. Some indoor allergens have an intermediate or indeterminant pattern of eliciting skin symptoms. Skin reactions from indoor allergens may also result from consuming or taking food, medicaments, or syrups that are contaminated with a particular allergen. A food allergen reaction may occur if food is eaten that contains oat or a medication that contains peanuts.

Indoor allergies can cause a variety of uncomfortable symptoms. The most common symptoms are sneezing, nasal congestion, a runny nose, or postnasal drip. These respiratory symptoms can cause a tickly throat, itchiness in the mouth, throat, and inner ear, and an ear infection if the Eustachian tube becomes obstructed, which may cause ear popping or fullness. People with allergic asthma who have the insurance of hay fever experience worsened asthma symptoms. Chronic postnasal drip may also result in a chronic cough, irritation in the throat, hoarseness, or difficulty speaking.

2. Pets as Indoor Allergy Triggers

Pets, especially pet dander, can be triggers for indoor allergies. In living spaces, dogs and especially cats sometimes may dwell. Regardless of a pet's shedding practices, their skin flakes are very tiny and easily airborne, which is why they are still an allergen source. They can be found in rugs, bedding, furniture, ventilation systems, and on just about any surface pet dander can settle. Ear and hair follicle exudates, urine, and feces produced by cats and dogs are released. Besides dander, these also contain allergen proteins. There are also that are similar. Individuals found to be allergic to one of these commonly turn out to be allergic to both. Cats' saliva contains a small protein. It sticks to cat fur when a cat licks herself or another one and dries. Similarly, all cats can potentially produce this type of allergen. The only cat that will not produce this allergen is one that is hairless. Since the hairless cat will still lick itself and other cats, some individuals are allergic to hairless cats. There are also allergens that are individual and specific to each cat. Cat allergen from saliva and all other cat allergens in general originate from the skin. Blood allergen levels are predictive of developing asthma in cat allergen-sensitized children.

2.1. Types of Pet Allergens

There are many types of pet allergens that cat and dog allergens produce, and each of these can produce one or more allergenic particles that partition into the home. Table 1 shows the potential allergen secretions produced by cats and dogs in the home that develop from the route of synthesis in the glandular cell to the full allergen to be considered by the homeowner. For most homes, those that permit pets within or on a person, there will be some secretory production of allergens into the home. Multi-pet and single-pet homes may differ because of the different amount of allergen that can be produced.

Unlike outdoor allergens that are distributed into the environment, pet allergens are internal ambient contaminants. Cats and dogs shed and secrete a wide range of allergenic proteins and glycoproteins, and some secrete less allergenic features such as size fragments and/or following binding to airborne particles. These features also partition through indoor reservoirs over time. The range of molecular structures suggests that some potent and ultra-potent allergens are emerging as well. Overall, such allergenic proteins and their structural and functional relationships form effective targets for preventing or treating allergic responses by directly attacking effects induced on mast cells of the allergic response. These allergens, and any allergenic proteases, also need to be considered as biotic factors that are potential contributors to and mediators of 'sick' building syndromes. Such information on allergens also suggests practical regimens that can reduce pollen, pet, and dust mite allergens, which should help to reduce risks of the allergy triangle in asthma and hay fever.

2.2. Strategies for Managing Pet Allergies

As home allergens, pet allergens are of two types – secretions in the form of tiny particles that fill the air as the animal moves. Not everyone is allergic to pets. Keeping a pet that you are allergic to is your decision; this guide offers you advice on minimizing the effects of pets on your health and business environment should you choose to keep the pet. Remember, parting with a pet that has been a household member for a number of years is challenging. Before you get a pet, it is important to ask your healthcare provider about pet allergies. For the family, there may be some pets that will not induce an allergic response. Always bear in mind that an allergy may develop to a pet that has been in the family for a long time.

It should be noted that strategies should be in place to curb exacerbation of allergy or asthma and make the inside of homes or work areas as friendly as possible. Our goal here is to set forth practical steps you can take to minimize the effects of pet allergens in your home, even if you own a pet.

2.2. Pets. Ah, pets. When it comes to pets, people typically talk about dogs and cats, but birds, rabbits, gerbils, guinea pigs, ferrets, and hamsters can also be classified as pets. Unlike pests, we typically choose pets.

3. Mold: Identification and Remediation

If visible mold is found in a home, an investigation by a certified or licensed mold inspector may be helpful in thoroughly identifying all potential sources of growth. To prevent mold growth in areas of water damage, it is often necessary to cut out and remove sections of contaminated or water-damaged materials. Because mold infiltration can carry risks if not appropriately managed, it is important to avoid do-it-yourself solutions. Qualified mold professionals can also advise on effective cleaning solutions if an HVAC or dust system needs to be cleaned or whether any surfaces need to be treated with bleach or another mold-killing product. When mold consulting is not available, low-odor, hypoallergenic cleansers or home remedies such as vinegar may be used after any visible mold growth has been physically removed. To prevent accidental inhalation and adverse health effects, individuals should wear personal protective equipment, such as masks, gloves, and goggles, when vacuuming, cleaning, or removing mold-affected materials.

Mold is one of the most pervasive indoor allergens. It is, however, sometimes difficult to locate and identify. Some common places to find mold in a home environment include damp floors, walls, or ceilings; wood cabinets, furniture, or floors; damp wood under carpet; walls behind furniture where condensation has formed; and the underside of sinks in cabinets where plumbing leaks have occurred. To prevent the growth of mold in homes, it is critical to control indoor humidity. A relative humidity of 30-50 percent is considered by many experts to be an important threshold that should not be exceeded in the management of mold or other indoor allergens. Dehumidifiers, mold-resistant paint, mold-control cleaners, and air purifiers are just a few examples of tools that can be used to keep mold in check within a residence.

3.1. Signs of Mold in the Home

Here are a few signs to be alert for if you suspect mold is present in your home. A musty or moldy odor is often noted when mold is present. This odor can be similar to the smell of feet or socks left to absorb sweat. Unrealistic odorous signs of mold in property may have been perceived by some mold victims to include, but are not limited to, cigar smoke, witches' brew, rotting vegetation, and dirt. Moreover, visual forms of mold are often visible and may appear as black or dark-colored mold and/or as a thin, thick, circular cluster of mold. Mold grows in places where significant water has been present.

Mold is a fungus that is found everywhere, both outside and inside. Various types of mold can grow in your home due to moisture, and being exposed to the allergens or irritants in mold can cause health problems. It has been well documented that mold exposure can have an array of human health complications, including, but not limited to, triggering allergic diseases such as allergic rhinitis, asthma, and atopic dermatitis. Signs of mold or mold exposure include respiratory symptoms such as a stuffy or runny nose and itchy, watery eyes, depressive signs, fever, or chills. Thus, it is very important that the first step to the reduction of indoor mold allergen is to manage mold in the home.

3.2. Methods for Mold Removal

Current evidence does not support the use of antimicrobial paints and wall coverings. In general, the dilutional and disruptive agents such as scrubbing and vacuuming are more effective than immobilization agents, such as encapsulation. developed a cleaning protocol that achieved substantial - greater than 90% - removal of Aspergillus, Penicillium, and Stachybotrys from survey plates used to compare cleaning methods. Using interviews with mold remediation workers, also found that damp wiping was most effective as a general cleaning method.

Mold removal from indoor environments should be done using both professional and do-it-yourself methods. The United States Environmental Protection Agency (EPA) guidelines suggest considering professional assistance if the mold is covering more than 10 square feet of area, if there is internal water damage or contaminants in the HVAC system, or if the water has been standing for more than two days. There are several strategies that can be used for mold removal. These strategies involve using detergents, water, and physical disturbance to remove soils from surfaces, as well as water to rinse the detergent and soil away. Some strategies are also intended to kill mold spores using biocides, with the intent of not only removing existing mold but also preventing future mold growth. Physical restraint methods such as encapsulation are intended to prevent future mold growth by altering physical access to the contaminants that the mold feeds on or by capturing the airborne spores in a film of resin.

4. Dust: A Persistent Indoor Allergen

Carpets, draperies, and upholstery in furniture provide a habitat for the mites, preventing allergy patients from effective environmental control. Reducing dust to control mites is the most effective protection measure. On the other hand, the protein allergen (mites and cockroaches) can dry up and float through the air when the relative humidity is too low as volatile particles, adhering to duct surfaces and increasing the allergy risk as they float back into the breathable air. These allergens can be removed from indoor surfaces, another important control method that helps prevent allergies by removing allergens.

Dust is found throughout the home, but its prevalence in bedding generates frequent allergic symptoms in the morning. Regrettably, our bodies produce flaky bedding that ejects dust and serves as a food source for mites. A mixture of mites, their body parts, and the waste they produce contain most of the major dust allergens. It has been suggested that one infested mattress may contain up to ten million mites or more.

Dust is one of the most common and persistent indoor allergens in a home. It is also one of the most challenging to control, as it exists indoors all year long and represents a mixture of a range of different substances. Among them are bacteria, food particles, mold spores, textiles, and dead skin. If not properly addressed, these items can serve as food for mites, themselves an important dust allergen.

4.1. Sources of Dust in the Home

A vacuum often promotes the removal of large and small dust flakes, which are the result of human skin construction and natural shedding. The amount of these large and small dust particles can range from a grain of salt to the width of a dog's hair. When cleaning, a vacuum will collect dust from windows, doors, walls, and other dust-retaining areas. If windows are opened for any length of time, additional sources of dust may infiltrate the environment. For most homeowners, the only method to minimize allergenic dust is to clean and vacuum on a regular basis. Varied levels of cleanliness will help to maintain down the overall amount of dust in the home, preventing larger particles from entering the air.

People are keenly interested in the things in their environment that are affecting their health, comfort, budget, and even peace of mind. The true sources of dust in homes are not well known by those outside of the indoor air quality industry. To hold on to some privacy and homeowner confidentiality, this lack of awareness is untold. But to properly inventory allergenic particles in a home, a general knowledge of potential dust developers is sometimes necessary. Because a lot of the below items need to be touched by several individuals in a home in the course of a day, we can deduce that these items will contribute to the amount of dust circulation within the home. These countless sources of dust and their expanding particles make it difficult for a homeowner to vacuum them and remove them from their home. As a result, we employ a strong filtering vacuum for the practice.

4.2. Tips for Dust Mite Control

- Pillows: Wash pillows every week in hot water in the washing machine. - Bedding: Wash sheets and blankets in hot water. - Stuffed toys: Limit the number of stuffed toys in the bed to one special friend. Wash in hot water or freeze toys to kill mites. - Carpets and rugs: Keep carpets and rugs out of your home. Dust collects in them and is hard to remove. If you do have carpet, make sure it is freshly vacuumed and vacuum at least three times per week using a vacuum with a HEPA filter cleaner and a double-layered microfilter bag. - Cleaning: Wipe the dust off surfaces and wash floors with a damp mop. Use a special allergen reducing cleaner. - Bedroom: Do not keep clutter – like newspapers – around the bed. Dust collects in clutter. - Windows: Keep the windows closed on windy days when there is a lot of pollen outside. - Outside: Have a low pollen yard. - Check the insulation. If insulation in the attic or crawl space is exposed, cover or have it professionally treated to decrease exposure.

While it is impossible to totally get rid of dust mites, there are some things you can do to reduce the number of dust mites in your home. It's very important to work on these changes even if you or your child does not show signs of allergies or asthma. These steps can help everyone stay healthy. Here are some tips to help control dust mites:

4. Use a vacuum cleaner equipped with a high efficiency particulate air filter (HEPA) and a double-layered microfilter bag to trap the tiniest dust mite allergens.

Special vacuum cleaners "seal" the area they are vacuuming so that the dust and other sucked items do not come back out into the room.

3. For stuffed animals, limit the number in your child's room. Launder stuffed toys in hot water or place them in a plastic bag in the freezer once a month for 24 hours to kill dust mites.

2. Wash your sheets and comforters every week in hot water that is at least 140°F. Drying the bedclothes in the dryer makes them even less appealing to dust mites. You may also want to wash curtains, soft toys, pet beds, and blankets once a week. If you cannot wash these items, you can also place them into a hot dryer for 15 minutes on the highest setting or if you can freeze them, at 0°F for 24 hours.

1. Cover pillows, mattress, and box springs in zippered dust mite proof covers. They are made of a thick, tightly woven fabric that keeps the dust mites and their tiny feces away from your face while you sleep.

5. Cleaning Supplies and Indoor Allergies

What types of allergens are found in cleaning products? Some of the common allergens found in cleaning supplies include fragrances, preservative chemicals, solvents, and ammonia, bleach, and preservatives. These allergens are known to cause asthma attacks. Therefore, for someone with allergies can trigger asthma. This is due to the VOCs (volatile organic compounds) found in the cleaning solutions. VOCs are released as gases and can contribute to exposure to indoor pollutants. The use of cleaning products then creates allergens and pollutants. This can lead to some people getting sick. An indoor allergy can cause skin rash, itchy eyes, sore throat, and shortness of breath. Yikes! This is why we always recommend everyone use green cleaners. They have natural ingredients including essential oils and vinegar. They clean well and are better for your health. Additionally, after using a harsh cleaning product, there are still microbes around causing allergens. That's why we have to spray a green cleaner and wipe the surfaces clean. We love Force of Nature because it cleans and works on surfaces. You can make your own cleaners as well.

Unlike what many people believe, cleaning supplies can be one of the reasons for experiencing indoor allergies. That's why it's important to use cleaning supplies that are free of harsh chemicals to eliminate your risks of getting indoor allergens that can be harmful to you and your family. Let's find out why and how you can do this.

5.1. Common Allergens in Cleaning Products

The most effective strategy to avoid these allergens is to use products that can be classified as standard cleaners & degreasers. However, standard cleaners & degreasers often contain both preservatives and fragrances. The chemicals examined range from concrete additives to water repellents, pigments, preservatives, and detergents. There are also multiple options for close chemical substitutions available on the market in many cases. To our knowledge, these chemicals have not been studied as allergy triggers or in any other way that would provide them with a special trade secret status and justify their inclusion in the confidential business information section.

It is challenging for allergic consumers to identify common allergens in a product on a pre-purchase basis. Until legislators provide allergen labeling mandates, an understanding of common allergens in each product group is vital for allergic individuals to make better product choices, thereby reducing their risk of an allergic reaction. The goal of this study was to distinguish and prioritize ingredients in cleaning products most commonly associated with allergy. The study focused on the six most common allergens that are believed to trigger indoor allergies, and thus lead to indoor allergy symptoms. Findings show that masks are the most cited source of indoor allergy triggers and a common recommendation to avoid them is to use cleaning products that do not contain certain listed allergens. We identify twelve known allergens for which avoidance could be beneficial in reducing consumer exposure to indoor allergy triggers by avoiding cleaning products that contain them as ingredients.

5.2. Alternative Cleaning Solutions

Of course, there are only so many times that a person can be expected to cycle linens in the laundry each week and carry out the necessary cleaning. "Afresh" washing machine tablets have been found to effectively remove built-up biofilm lurking in the dark, moist recesses of a front load or top load washing machine that may add bioburden on the fabrics put through a wash cycle. Afresh washing machine tablets designed for an empty machine cycle are run as a full machine of 5-6 cleaning tablets where water is added and diluted with a tablet's cleaning material over a 36-minute wash cycle. Following your first 'Afresh' washing machine tablet run, this must be repeated the following three weeks.

Effective cleaning strategies are essential for minimizing indoor allergy triggers in the world. The five biggest must-haves for an allergen-free interior that must be regularly cleaned include pillows, sheets, window treatments, clothing, and pets. The data suggests that washing these triggers every week is necessary to reduce allergen levels. Also, making sure that the air diffuser directs air away from these collection areas that house these triggers can be powerful. According to the previous data, an air diffuser located directly above a bed with linens in place can create an unintentional mixing chamber where air from an air diffuser disrupts collected allergen, leading to a spiky cloud of allergen over the bed days later. Avoid using ceiling fans or any kind of power air diffusing device that stirs up the micro-contaminants in a room.

6. Creating an Allergy-Friendly Home Environment

While proper allergy treatment can aid in managing allergy symptoms, the importance of reducing allergens in our environment, upholding indoor air quality and the allergy-friendliness of our homes are key. Dust mites, pet dander, and other allergy triggers can affect a person's health. In many cases, doctors will recommend making changes at home. The following strategies can help control allergens and improve air quality. Regular cleaning can reduce allergen levels. A few sensitive tools include vacuum cleaners and dehumidifiers. Plain tap water is more effective than dusting. Because the dust does not fly in the air, the bed microparticles dry with the mules. Dust removal will not get rid of the dust. A HEPA (high-efficiency particulate air) filter can trap irritating particles. Look for a vacuum cleaner or air purifier that has a HEPA filter. Prior to a visit, it may help less fragrance, less deodorant, and less sniff.

The Environmental Protection Agency is least likely to be allergic to us at the bottom of any inhaled allergens that hold earlier than were amateur! One reason for this change is that many of the medications that are now on the market because they are similar to the medications in many of today's medical communities most often prescribed that have been dispensed at higher dosages and are still delivered to the patient. Another reason for these drugs is to help create resistance to the disease so that the doctor will not be worried about the seriousness of the medicine used medications. With the lower limits of medicine, prescription companies are spending money and resources trying to heal this deadly disease with clean money. This last year we added a daily adipic so that our indoor air quality would be cleaned and because we liked to smoke groceries odor, it also made us healthy. The water remains so distilled that the animals drink in abundance, and everyone is a winner;)

6.1. Importance of Indoor Air Quality

In the United States, most individuals spend around 90% of their life indoors, so it is imperative for their well-being that the environment they inhabit is safe and healthy. Poor indoor air quality can lead to the following non-allergic as well as allergic symptoms: eye irritation, headaches, fatigue, lethargy, shortness of breath, sinus congestion, coughing, skin rashes, asthma attacks, infections, hives, and upper respiratory congestion. Research has shown that adults, children, and infants are all at risk for developing medical problems that are associated with poor indoor air quality. Adult women are at a higher risk than adult men for developing infection, pneumonia, and pulmonary diseases as a result of inadequate indoor air quality. In addition, newborns, who breathe approximately 50% more air per pound of body weight, and young children, who are more physically active and do not always make smart food and drink choices, are more vulnerable to sickness and experiencing side effects from exposure to pollutants.

Indoor air quality plays an essential role in the management of indoor allergies. Substances such as dust mite, animal and cockroach particles, and mold spores are notorious for causing allergic reactions, triggering symptoms such as a stuffy or runny nose, sneezing, itchy or watery eyes, and exacerbated asthma. Luckily, there are several strategies individuals can use to manage their exposure to these indoor allergens to lessen their indoor allergies. While symptoms caused by exposure to outdoor environmental allergens (such as pollens, molds, and fungi) can also be addressed, overall, the efficacy of these treatments can increase when individuals manage indoor allergen exposure. Through evidence-based research, this guide provides an overview of steps to manage indoor allergen exposure that can result in reduced symptoms and improved quality of life.

6.2. Tips for Reducing Allergens in the Home

Focus dust mite reduction efforts on a patient's sleep space—and don't forget to check underneath the bed. Encase the mattress, box spring, and pillows in a material designed to keep dust mites from taking up residence. Set the water heater to 130°F. This can kill dust mites and their eggs. "High heat and water make steam, which can reduce dust mites," Dr. Selcow says. "If it is handled properly, not only will dust mites die, but you're getting rid of the mold spores as well." Be sure to place soft toys or dolls in the dryer as well if they can tolerate heat. If a stuffed animal can't tolerate being washed, place them in the freezer overnight. The cold will kill the dust mites. Periodically dust the headboard and any other shelving near the bed, and vacuum around the bed. "People forget to clean nine inches under the bed," Dr. Selcow says, "But that's where dust mites primarily come from."

• With Dust Mites, Up Is Down

Everyone knows that managing allergies means avoiding triggers. To create an indoor environment that's more allergy-friendly, patients need to reduce irritants, such as dust mites, pet dander, or mold spores, which can lead to symptoms. While it's impossible to remove all allergy triggers, an allergist can help patients find ways to limit their exposure, which can help lessen symptoms. But some common advice may actually make things worse. Mention these things to consider.

• Better Management Begins at Home

7. Conclusion and Future Directions

In conclusion, aside from allergen avoidance strategies, allergen-specific immunotherapy also exists to change the immune response to the allergen by down-regulating the allergic response to the allergen and increasing tolerance. However, ASIT is not included in our current review, and we did not relieve prescribed medication for patients with allergies. Several emerging technologies have been recently developed for the management of indoor allergies and, in particular, appeal to the end user with smart technologies including mobile phone apps and tracking devices. Emerging products are often focused on animal allergen management and were not reviewed. Further research could directly compare the commercially attractive end user products, such as smart products currently in development, to determine how effective they are, what the research limitations may be (e.g., selection bias from self-selection), and which areas may be researched further to assist in their viability as a solution.

In summary, the previous three chapters reviewed several strategies for managing indoor allergens. The basic strategies are to eliminate or reduce allergen exposure by altering the indoor environment. The most common strategy is the use of house dust mite impermeable encasements. However, other strategies have shown mixed results. For example, there are differing opinions regarding the use of carpeting in the home. The use of air purifiers and dehumidifiers has also shown mixed results. The use of barrier bedding, electrostatic air filters, and filter vacuums have shown no clear benefit in a multi-center trial. Multifaceted comprehensive allergen management strategies that use a combination of different control measures and pharmacologic treatments are more successful. However, these strategies are more complex and cost more to implement. A more recent strategy for preventing allergic diseases, specifically asthma, is to change diet and supplementation in neonates (breastfeeding vs formula) and during pregnancy and discuss probiotic supplements. While a small number of studies mention these strategies, the data are not reviewed here. Considering the results of this review, the challenges for indoor allergen management are to design effective solutions that are affordable and sustainable. Further research should prioritize the comparison of commercially available products and those still in the development stage.

7.1. Summary of Key Strategies

The benefits of these four main strategies are cumulative because by practicing as many of these strategies as possible, the amount of allergenic particulate indoors and in the air can be kept to a minimum. Changing the furnishings and one's lifestyle will not cure the cause of allergic diseases, but it will reduce the allergen intake in symptomatic individuals. Fewer useful and effective allergen avoidance measures are available for outdoor allergens. Major sources of outdoor allergens include pollen and fungal spores. Because of their small size, these allergens are usually found suspended in outdoor air. The four main strategies are highly effective in managing indoor allergens.

The only complete solution for managing dust mites, as well as many other indoor allergens, is to improve the quality of the indoor air by reducing the concentration of inhaled allergens. To achieve this goal, there are four strategies to consider. The first main strategy is to prevent the entry of outdoor allergens into indoor environments. The second main strategy is to maintain the relative humidity in indoor environments at an optimal level that deters the growth of mites and molds. The third strategy is to remove the food source of mites, animal dander, and molds from indoor environments, and the fourth strategy is to remove or inactivate the sources of indoor allergens. Because much of the responsibility for keeping the allergens out of the lungs falls on the room air, the first three strategies for managing indoor allergens are described here, whereas the fourth strategy is outlined in Section III.

7.2. Emerging Technologies for Allergy Management

Emerging technologies are needed that can foster a reactive and effective built environment capable of delivering personal environments that do not exacerbate asthma or allergies. Instead of only treating the allergy ex post facto, or judging allergic individuals for their actions, for example, we could create intelligent homes that could sense pollen levels and open and close windows accordingly. Rather than hoping all residents have learned the correct set of propagandized attitudes, we could create preemptive built environments that function with personal appliances to achieve indoor air quality management collective, behaving very differently during an alert of a nearby upwind wildfire. Addressing these problems of requirements, of device capacities, and of logical capacities is a challenge, but it is also an opportunity, and one with potential for reducing inequality in the lived experience of sensitive individuals and breaking down boundaries that prevent full participation in the built environment.

Allergy management has come a long way since static electricity conditioning, let alone since before the advent of centrally heated and cooled structures. An allergy-free home can do a world of good for caregiving and independence, and effective indoor allergy management is crucial. We have discussed medications, filtration, ventilation, humidity control, education strategies, barriers, off-site management, and professionally managed approaches for addressing a range of indoor allergy triggers in the built environment. Nonetheless, there are further strides to be made, and beyond the sheer performance of such devices, there is a concomitant range of other issues to consider, from ease of use to economic costs to human factors such as attitudes towards this embodied environmental control.